Transport Statistics Repo

GW00372453

5·941

Cars : Make and Model : The Risk of Driver Injury and Car Accident Rates in Great Britain : 1994

November 1995

London: HMSO

Prepared for publication by STD5 Branch
Directorate of Statistics
Department of Transport

Jeremy Grove
Peter Wilding

GOVERNMENT STATISTICAL SERVICE

A service of statistical information and advice is provided to
the government by specialist staff employed in the statistics
divisions of individual Departments. Statistics are made
generally available through their publications and further
information and advice on them can be obtained from the
Departments concerned.

Enquiries about the contents of this publication should be
made to:

Directorate of Statistics
Department of Transport
Room B649
Romney House
43 Marsham Street
London SW1P 3PY

Telephone 071-276-8780

Contents

INTRODUCTION

This publication presents estimates of the risk of driver injury in popular models of car once involved in a two car collision injury accident. It also includes, at a more general level, estimates of accident involvement rates and associated casualty rates analysed, within broad groups, by age and performance of car, and whether the car is privately or company owned. The statistics in this publication are based on personal injury road accident data reported to the Department of Transport by police forces within Great Britain.

The publication is in three parts:

Part 1 The risk of driver injury in popular models of car once involved in two car collision injury accidents, generally known as secondary or passive safety. Estimates are shown in Tables A and B.

Part 2 Car accident involvement and casualty rates, generally known as primary or active safety. Estimates are shown in Tables C and D.

Part 3 Summaries of other related work which has been carried out by the Department.

Structural design is the key factor in secondary safety and is complemented by good design of interior fittings, particularly seat belts, energy absorbing steering wheels and columns, padded dashboards and the provision of airbag supplementary restraints. Together these have great potential for reducing the number of road casualties. By contrast, primary safety - accident avoidance - is mainly influenced by the driver but vehicle design features such as good braking, handling, stability, lighting and driver vision, can all help the driver to avoid accidents.

The first part of the publication summarises the adopted methodology which uses the risk of driver injury as a basis for assessing the secondary safety features of cars, sets out the results in Tables A and B, and summarises the main conclusions. The second part of the publication summarises the accident involvement and casualty rates for particular groups of car, sets out results in Tables C and D, and summarises the main conclusions. The third part outlines progress on work on calculating car safety ratings which only reflect inherent structural safety and the efficiency of safety fittings by excluding the effect of mass in an injury accident. There is also an examination of the aggressivity of cars in injury accidents. This has been determined as the risk of injury to the other driver involved in a collision with a certain model of car. It also includes an analysis of factors affecting the severity of injury to pedestrians hit by cars. This is followed by a section in the form of appendices which set out definitions, and a more detailed description of the source and coverage of the car accident data used in this report for the estimation of car driver injury accident rates.

PART 1

SECONDARY CAR SAFETY (Tables A and B)

Measuring Secondary Car Safety

1.1   One approach for assessing secondary car safety is to simulate typical accidents by crashing a car into a fixed block under controlled conditions and, in some cases, to measure the forces on dummy occupants. Such crash tests are able to control the severity of accident and assess the secondary safety design effects in a simulated collision. The shortcoming of these types of test is that they are representative of only some real life collisions.

1.2   Another approach to measuring secondary safety is to look at real life injury accident data. This is a more complicated approach because, unlike crash tests where severity of accident can be controlled, severity of real-life accidents can be highly variable which makes it difficult to compare injury data for different car models. This is because different car models may be exposed to different types of accident and may be driven predominantly by different groups of drivers.

1.3   The measure of secondary safety for popular models of cars in this publication is based upon the risk of driver injury in two-car injury accidents. This is a relatively straightforward calculation because in every injury accident it is known whether the driver is injured or uninjured because every car must have a driver, except for parked cars which are not included in the analysis. A fuller measure of secondary car safety could also include the risk of injury to front seat passengers. However this is not so straightforward to calculate because only information on injured passengers is recorded by the police, and any risk calculation would have to be based on assumptions about the average number of front seat passengers in models of car to which the number of injured front seat passengers could be compared. Since average front seat occupancy is likely to be variable in different models of car, it was decided to measure secondary safety on the narrower but more reliable definition of driver injury only.

1.4   An assessment of the relative risk of injury in different car models will also be influenced by their rate of involvement in non-injury, ie. damage-only, accidents. However, this analysis is necessarily constrained by the availability of only injury accident data.

1.5   In this section, for any injury accident involving a particular model of car, the risk of driver injury is expressed as the proportion of injury accidents in which drivers of that model are injured. These proportions, or rates, are relative rates in the sense that in any two car collision, the relative risk of driver injury not only depends upon the protection offered by the car being driven but also the safety performance of the car being hit. Most popular models of car tend to collide with a similar range of other cars in two car collisions, so for each model the risk of driver injury in that model is being assessed relative to the same average level of safety offered by injury accident involved cars.

1.6   An interesting point to note is the influence of interior, as distinct from exterior, secondary safety features upon the risk of injury in, say, two car collisions. If only one of the cars in a two car collision is fitted with an interior secondary safety device (such as an airbag) then the relative risk of driver injury in that car will be lower. If one of the cars in a two car collision is fitted with better exterior safety devices (such as superior energy absorbing bumpers or crumple zones) the relative risk of injury to both drivers in that particular collision is not affected, since the benefit of these devices is shared equally by both cars. However over the whole range of accidents the beneficial effects upon the risk of driver injury will be relatively concentrated on those models fitted with a superior exterior secondary safety device.

1.7   In this publication, the risk of driver injury in an injury accident provides the basis for assessing the protection that a car offers its driver. The main methodological problem in comparing driver injury risk in different cars is that the risks are influenced not only by the cars' safety features, but also by the severity of each of the individual accidents in which they are involved. The average severity of accident for each model will be influenced not only by the types of accident they are involved in, but also by the type of driver group which predominates in a particular model of car. For example, some cars may be involved in relatively more injury accidents on motorways at higher speeds than other cars, and some may be driven more by women whose risk of injury once involved in an accident is higher than that for men. A recent study by Dr Jeremy Broughton at the Transport Research Laboratory "The theoretical basis for comparing the accident record of car models" (see References in Appendix 1) confirmed the broad extent to which different models of car are driven by different groups of driver and are involved in accidents different types of road (built-up or non built-up roads).

1.8   Only accidents involving two car collisions are considered in the assessment of car secondary safety in order to minimise distortions to the estimates of driver injury risk arising, for example, from a particular model of car having a high proportion of collisions with very large mass vehicles such as Goods Vehicles or Public Service Vehicles. Within the two car accident dataset there will still be some bias in the estimates of driver injury risk for each car model because of the different types of accident and driver involvement for some models of car. These influences are allowed for in a modelling procedure described in Appendix 3. In fact the adjustments made to estimates of driver injury risk to allow for these sources of bias are quite small. Nevertheless the adjusted estimates are the best estimates of secondary car safety derived from the two car collision dataset, and reflect the benefit of the secondary safety protection offered to the driver of a particular car, as well as the benefit of the size or mass of that car.

1.9   In addition to speed a major influence on the severity of accident is the mass of the car. In any two car collision the greater the mass of one of the cars involved in the collision the lower the deceleration force and risk of driver injury in that car. However in that same collision the deceleration force and risk of driver injury in the other lower mass car will usually be higher. Although mass provides safety benefits for the driver of a high mass car it also increases the risk of driver injury in those cars in collision with high mass cars.

1.10   In general, mass and size of car are closely related. In larger cars there is usually more room for crumple zones which absorb energy and reduce deceleration forces upon the driver and occupants, reducing their risk of injury. However, unlike mass, this feature of larger cars can also benefit the occupants of cars they collide with.

1.11   Most models of car collide with a similar size distribution of other cars. Appendix 4 shows the distribution of collisions for each model in relation to the mass group of the other car involved in the collision. At this level of aggregation the distributions are very similar. This leads to the conclusion that in two car accidents a safety rating for each model is calculated as if each car had collided with a car of average mass.

1.12   The rates shown in Table A retain for each particular model the effect of mass as a safety factor. A high mass car, apart from mostly offering more protection to its driver than a small mass car, can also appear to be safer in the statistical rates because it relatively increases the risk of injury in the car that it collides with. Heavy cars are likely to be more aggressive to other cars involved in the collision than light cars, although structural design is also an important factor. The fact that the risk of driver injury is lower in a higher mass car, but that the risk of injury in the other car involved in the collision is higher, presents an interesting paradox. The ratings shown in Table A reflect the benefit of mass to the driver; Part 3 describes a method for assessing a car's safety after allowance has been made for the influence of mass upon the risk of driver injury. This, in principle, removes the benefit of mass from the calculation of the risk of driver injury, so that derivative safety ratings for different models are based on their design, and the effectiveness of their safety fittings, rather than their mass.

1.13   In Table A cars have been classified into four size groups. Within each of the size groups the variation in mass between cars will be less than the variation in mass between cars in different size groups. This means that the risk of driver injury in cars of broadly similar mass within each size group can be compared to assess the protection offered by the structure and design of the car and its secondary safety fittings. But even within the four size groups there remains some mass variation.

Table A : Description

1.14   Table A sets out estimates of the risk of driver injury in two car driver injury accidents, for particular models of car, in four size groups, broadly defined by length of car. The estimates are based on accidents involving two cars during the years 1989 to 1994 inclusive. Ratings are only published for cars first registered on or after 1st January 1985. The rating for all sizes of car includes those models for which results are not presented individually while the size group averages are based on a weighted average of those models listed in the respective group. The calculation of the risk as the percentage of drivers injured in a specific model of car (say car 1) when involved in an injury accident with any other car (say car 2) can be represented schematically as follows:

$$\frac{X_1 + X_2}{X_1 + X_2 + X_3} \times 100$$

where

X_1 = Number of accidents in which driver injured in car 1 but not in car 2
X_2 = Number of accidents in which driver injured in car 1 and in car 2
X_3 = Number of accidents in which driver injured in car 2 but not in car 1

1.15   Within each size group (Small, Small/Medium, Medium, and Large) estimates are shown for each constituent model of car for all injuries and for fatal or serious injuries. The confidence intervals are also shown for each estimate for each car model. These show the range within which 95 per cent of the time the true rate will lie.

1.16   For both fatal or serious injuries and all injuries, uncorrected estimates (where no allowances have been made for types of accident or types of driver on the injury rates) are shown in brackets. The corrected estimates are shown alongside their respective confidence intervals. It can be seen that allowing for variation in the type of accidents and type of driver in specific car models does not have a great effect. However some of the allowances are only based on approximate indicators (speed of road as an indicator for speed of accident) and it may be that the available data are not sensitive enough to pick up such effects.

1.17   The estimates in Table A are based only on two car accidents, which has the benefit of directly eliminating the possibly distorting effects on the ratings, for some models of car, of a higher incidence of single vehicle accidents and collisions with large mass vehicles such as Goods Vehicles and Public Service Vehicles.

1.18   The most significant adjustment was for female drivers. Female drivers are more prone to injury for a given severity of accident and they tend to drive smaller cars than men. The main adjustment therefore tended to improve the uncorrected ratings for small cars where there was a higher incidence of women drivers, but to degrade the uncorrected ratings for large cars where there was a lower incidence of female drivers. Details of the adjustment process for driver influence and type of accident which influence severity of accident can be found in Appendix 3.

Table A : Commentary

1.19   The corrected best estimates of the percentage of drivers injured in any particular model, and their associated confidence intervals, can be used to assess which cars in any group are significantly different from the average risk for the group. Those models with a higher than average risk of driver injury offer a lower than average level of secondary protection, and vice versa for those models with a lower than average risk of driver injury. The estimates have been calculated after allowances have been made for the possible influence of exposure to different types of accident and driver. The specific influences that were looked at were age and sex of driver, point of impact, and speed limit of road as an indicator of severity of accident. More models are identified as being statistically different from their relevant group average for all injuries than for fatal or serious injuries because of the much larger proportions in the samples for all injuries compared to fatal or serious injuries. Consequently the confidence intervals are relatively narrower for all injuries.

1.20   Particular car models can be said to be statistically different (95 per cent of the time) from their respective group average if that average lies outside the confidence interval for the particular model. For example, in the grouping of small size cars shown in Table A the Citroen 2CV/Dyane is statistically different from the average risk of driver injury (for all injuries) in all small cars since the confidence interval for the Citroen model (80 to 88 per cent) does not include the estimate of average risk in all small cars (71 per cent). Similarly differences between particular models can be identified if the respective confidence intervals do not overlap. For example, the confidence interval for the Citroen 2CV/Dyane (80 to 88 per cent) does not overlap with the confidence interval for the Renault Clio (61 to 69 per cent).

1.21   The four groups of car shown in Table A have been essentially determined by length of car. Within each of the groups the specific model groupings of car have been determined by considering production line information about specific car models to ensure that the model groupings consist of models with as uniform design as possible. There will be some variation in mass between car models in each of the size groups despite the attempt to standardise the size classification of the four car groups. The estimates of risk of injury for each car model within each size group will reflect variations in mass, and also the secondary safety design and fittings features offered by each model. The important effect of mass and size on injury risk is clearly shown in Table A. The average risk of injury falls steadily with group size from 71 per cent for small cars to 46 per cent for large cars, confirming that, generally, the greater the mass of the car the greater the safety benefit to the driver of that car involved in a collision. In addition, drivers of larger cars are more likely to benefit from more extensive crumple zones. However, it is also true that the greater the mass of the car, the higher the risk of injury in the car that it collides with. This aggressive disbenefit of mass is described further in Part 3 of the publication.

1.22   The four graphs following the commentary on Table A show the safety ratings for groups of car models within each of the four size groups. The safety rating is derived from the risk of injury shown in Table A and relates the risk of injury in a particular model of car to the risk of injury in the overall average car. For example the rating for the Volvo 300 (small/medium cars) is calculated as follows:

All Injury risk (Volvo 300) best estimate $\qquad$ = 55%

All Injury risk (Overall Average car) best estimate = 62%

$$\text{Safety Rating} = \frac{62\% - 55\%}{62\%} \times 100 = +11\%$$

1.23   This shows that the safety rating for the Volvo 300, in terms of the statistical best estimate, is 11 per cent more than that for the overall average car. A similar calculation is carried out to show how the confidence interval for the safety rating, which includes the best estimate, relates to the overall average car, and these confidence intervals are shown in the four graphs. For example the confidence interval for the Volvo 300 shows that the estimate of the safety rating for this car could be between 8 and 15 per cent better than for the overall average car. The graphs show the confidence interval for each model's rating. Although the ratings have been calculated with reference to the overall average car, the graphs show them in relation to both the overall average and also their respective group average. Within each group of similar sized cars the graphs clearly show groups of cars which, at the 95 per cent level of confidence, are statistically different from their group average, and also from other models within the same group. The following table shows the distribution of these differences within each size group:

Car Size	Below Group Average	Around Group Average	Above Group Average	All Models
Small	5	15	2	22
Small/medium	6	20	10	36
Medium	4	16	9	29
Large	5	7	8	20
All	20	58	29	107

1.24   In each graph, make/models are presented alphabetically within the following three groups; models whose confidence intervals fall entirely below, around and entirely above the average for that size group. The effect of size and mass upon the ratings shows through when the confidence intervals are compared with the overall average. The intervals for small cars mostly fall below the overall average line, but the intervals for large cars all fall above the overall average line.

1.25   The 107 models listed in Table A include 19 examples where the model name has been retained by the manufacturer for a newer replacement model, but where the newer versions of that name include different design features and are therefore treated separately in the analysis. In several of these cases a series of three successive models appears in the tables. The replacement models generally provide at least as much protection to their drivers as their predecessors, and the latest versions of the following five models provide significantly better protection: Ford Escort, Nissan Micra, Rover 200/400, Vauxhall Astra, Vauxhall Cavalier. This pattern extends to the new versions of other models, and also to new models, for which ratings are also generally better than the average for their respective size groups.

Guide to make/models in graphs, and sample sizes [1]

Car size/model [2]	Registration dates	Number of involvements	Car size/model [2]	Registration dates	Number of involvements
SMALL			**MEDIUM**		
CITROEN 2CV/DYANE	Jan 85 - Jul 90 [3]	371	AUDI 80/90 A	Jan 85 - Oct 86	638
CITROEN AX	Jun 87 - Dec 94	1,764	AUDI 80/90 B	Nov 86 - Dec 94	683
CITROEN VISA	Jan 85 - Jul 88 [3]	251	BMW 3 SERIES A	Jan 85 - Mar 91	2,200
FIAT 126	Jan 85 - Dec 92	181	BMW 3 SERIES B	Apr 91 - Dec 94	420
FIAT PANDA	Jan 85 - Dec 94	1,538	CITROEN BX	Jan 85 - Dec 93 [3]	3,051
FIAT UNO	Jan 85 - Dec 94	3,333	FORD MONDEO	Mar 93 - Dec 94	602
FORD FIESTA A	Jan 85 - Mar 89	10,837	FORD SIERRA/SAPPHIRE	Jan 85 - Feb 93	15,330
FORD FIESTA B	Apr 89 - Dec 94	6,543	HONDA ACCORD A	Oct 85 - Sep 91	606
NISSAN MICRA A	Jan 85 - Dec 92	4,128	HONDA ACCORD B	Oct 91 - Jul 94	180
NISSAN MICRA B	Jan 93 - Dec 94	222	HONDA PRELUDE	Jan 85 - Mar 92	209
PEUGEOT 106	Oct 91 - Dec 94	486	HYUNDAI STELLAR	Jan 85 - Dec 91	298
PEUGEOT 205	Jan 85 - Dec 94	5,446	MAZDA 626 A	Jan 85 - Sep 87	268
RENAULT 5	Feb 85 - Dec 94	2,684	MAZDA 626 B	Oct 87 - Jan 92	350
RENAULT CLIO	Mar 91 - Dec 94	668	MERCEDES 190	Jan 85 - Sep 93	739
ROVER METRO A	Jan 85 - Mar 90	8,491	NISSAN BLUEBIRD	Mar 86 - Aug 90 [3]	3,023
ROVER METRO B	Apr 90 - Dec 94	1,704	NISSAN PRIMERA	Sep 90 - Dec 94	414
ROVER MINI	Jan 85 - Dec 94	1,690	PEUGEOT 405	Jan 88 - Dec 94	2,940
VAUXHALL CORSA	Mar 93 - Dec 94	393	RENAULT 21	Jun 86 - Mar 94	1,273
VAUXHALL NOVA	Jan 85 - Mar 93	5,905	ROVER MONTEGO	Jan 85 - Dec 94	5,354
VW POLO	Jan 85 - Aug 94	2,636	SUBARU 1.6/1.8	Jan 85 - Dec 91	201
YUGO 3/4/500	Jan 85 - Dec 91	171	TOYOTA CAMRY	Jan 85 - Dec 86	239
YUGO TEMPO	Jan 85 - Dec 93	428	TOYOTA CARINA EARLY	Jan 85 - Feb 88	326
			TOYOTA CARINA MID	Mar 88 - Apr 92	452
TOTAL [4]		102,510	TOYOTA CARINA E	May 92 - Dec 94	182
			VAUXHALL CAVALIER A	Jan 85 - Sep 88	5,614
			VAUXHALL CAVALIER B	Oct 88 - Dec 94	7,176
SMALL/MEDIUM			VW PASSAT/SANTANA	Jan 85 - May 88	390
			VW PASSAT	Jun 88 - Dec 94	500
ALFA ROMEO 33	Jan 85 - Dec 94	188	VOLVO 400	Jun 87 - Dec 94	806
CITROEN ZX	Jun 91 - Dec 94	504			
FIAT STRADA/REGATA	Jan 85 - Jun 88 [3]	517	TOTAL [4]		126,738
FIAT TIPO/TEMPRA	Jul 88 - Dec 94	735			
FORD ESCORT/ORION A	Jan 85 - Aug 90	23,728			
FORD ESCORT/ORION B	Sep 90 - Dec 94	4,355	**LARGE**		
HYUNDAI PONY	Oct 85 - Aug 90	406			
LADA RIVA [5]	Jan 85 - Dec 94	1,214	AUDI 100/200	Jan 85 - Dec 94	458
LADA SAMARA	Nov 87 - Dec 94	525	BMW 5 SERIES A	Jan 85 - May 88	428
LANCIA DELTA/PRISMA	Jan 85 - Jul 94	182	BMW 5 SERIES B	Jun 88 - Dec 94	633
MAZDA 323 A	Sep 85 - Sep 89	465	FIAT CROMA	Jun 86 - Dec 93 [3]	170
MAZDA 323 B	Oct 89 - Jul 94	264	FORD GRANADA	May 85 - Dec 94	2,824
NISSAN CHERRY	Jan 85 - Aug 86 [3]	529	JAGUAR XJ	Oct 86 - Dec 94	561
NISSAN SUNNY A	Jan 85 - Aug 86	753	MERCEDES S CLASS	Jan 85 - Sep 91	199
NISSAN SUNNY B	Sep 86 - Jan 91	2,110	MERCEDES 200/300	Oct 85 - Dec 94	682
NISSAN SUNNY C	Feb 91 - Dec 94	239	PEUGEOT 505	Jan 85 - Dec 91 [3]	266
PEUGEOT 305	Jan 85 - Jul 88 [3]	389	RENAULT 25	Jan 85 - Jan 93	695
PEUGEOT 306	Apr 93 - Dec 94	196	ROVER 800	Jul 86 - Dec 94	1,895
PEUGEOT 309	Feb 86 - Mar 93	3,079	ROVER SD1	Jan 85 - Jun 86 [3]	220
PROTON 1.3/1.5	Mar 89 - Dec 94	473	SAAB 900	Jan 85 - Sep 93	461
RENAULT 19	Feb 89 - Dec 94	1,011	SAAB 9000	Oct 85 - Dec 94	368
RENAULT 9/11	Jan 85 - Jan 89 [3]	957	VAUXHALL CARLTON A	Jan 85 - Oct 86	503
ROVER 200	Jan 85 - Sep 89	3,563	VAUXHALL CARLTON B	Nov 86 - Mar 94	1,548
ROVER 200/400	Oct 89 - Dec 94	2,791	VAUXHALL SENATOR	Sep 87 - Mar 94	385
ROVER MAESTRO	Jan 85 - Dec 94	3,691	VOLVO 200	Jan 85 - Dec 94	640
SEAT IBIZA/MALAGA	Oct 85 - Sep 93	715	VOLVO 700	Jan 85 - Jul 91 [3]	1,370
SKODA ESTELLE	Jan 85 - Jul 90 [3]	700	VOLVO 900	Oct 90 - Dec 94	220
SKODA FAVORIT	Jun 89 - Dec 94	241			
TOYOTA COROLLA A	Jan 85 - Aug 87	587	TOTAL [4]		26,418
TOYOTA COROLLA B	Sep 87 - Jul 92	858			
VAUXHALL ASTRA/BELMONT	Jan 85 - Sep 91	10,778			
VAUXHALL ASTRA	Oct 91 - Dec 94	1,619			
VW GOLF MK1/CABRIOLET	Jan 85 - Dec 93	653			
VW GOLF/JETTA	Jan 85 - Jan 92	4,620			
VW GOLF/VENTO	Feb 92 - Dec 94	494			
VOLVO 300	Jan 85 - Dec 91 [3]	2,222			
TOTAL [4]		98,113			

1 Number of involvements in two car collisions in which at least one driver was injured - the samples on which Table A and the graphs are based. Note that this number does not represent all accidents involving vehicles of the given model.

2 Models are listed under the current market name of the manufacturer.

3 Approximate withdrawal date. All cars registered up to December 1994 are included.

4 Totals include listed models, models whose sample size was insufficient and models whose first registration data is earlier than 1 January 1985.

5 Includes earlier 1200, 1300, 1500 and 1600 models.

Relative driver protection by make/model 1989-94
Small cars

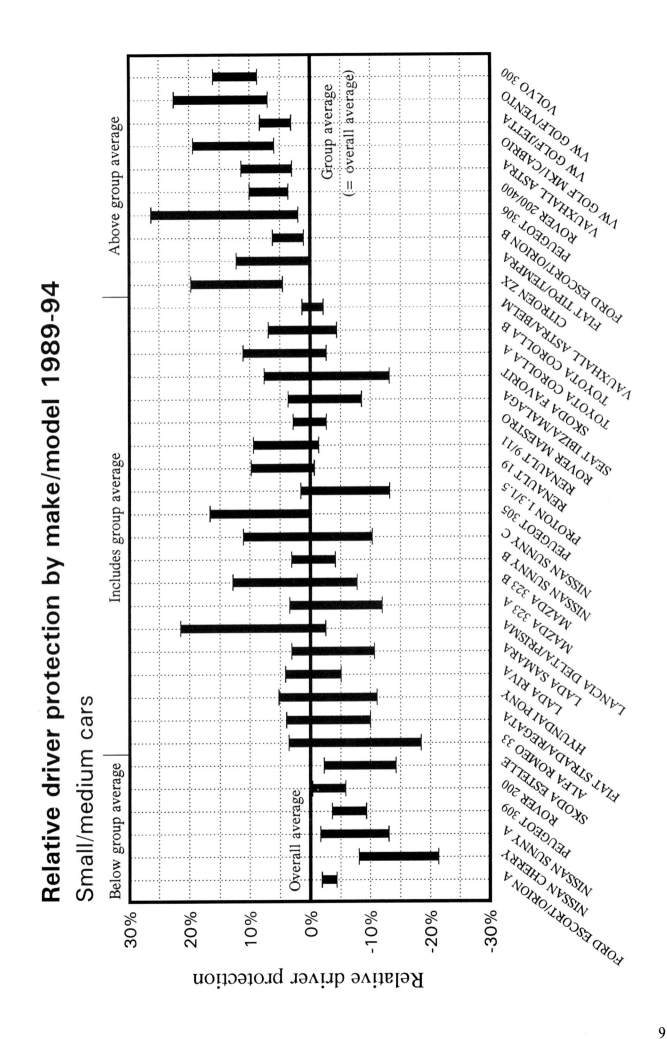

Relative driver protection by make/model 1989-94

Small/medium cars

Relative driver protection

30% — 20% — 10% — 0% — -10% — -20% — -30%

Above group average

Includes group average

Below group average

Group average
(= overall average)

Overall average

FORD ESCORT/ORION A
NISSAN CHERRY
PEUGEOT 309
ROVER 200
SKODA ESTELLE
ALFA ROMEO 33
FIAT STRADA/REGATA
HYUNDAI PONY
LADA RIVA
LANCIA DELTA/PRISMA
MAZDA 323 A
MAZDA 323 B
NISSAN SUNNY B
NISSAN SUNNY C
PEUGEOT 305
PROTON 1.3/1.5
RENAULT 19
ROVER MAESTRO
SEAT IBIZA/MALAGA
SKODA FAVORIT
TOYOTA COROLLA A
TOYOTA COROLLA B
VAUXHALL ASTRA/BELMONT
CITROEN ZX
FIAT TIPO/TEMPRA
FORD ESCORT/ORION B
PEUGEOT 306
ROVER 200/400
VAUXHALL ASTRA
VW GOLF MK1/CABRIO
VW GOLF/JETTA
VW GOLF/VENTO
VOLVO 300

9

Relative driver protection by make/model 1989-94

Medium cars

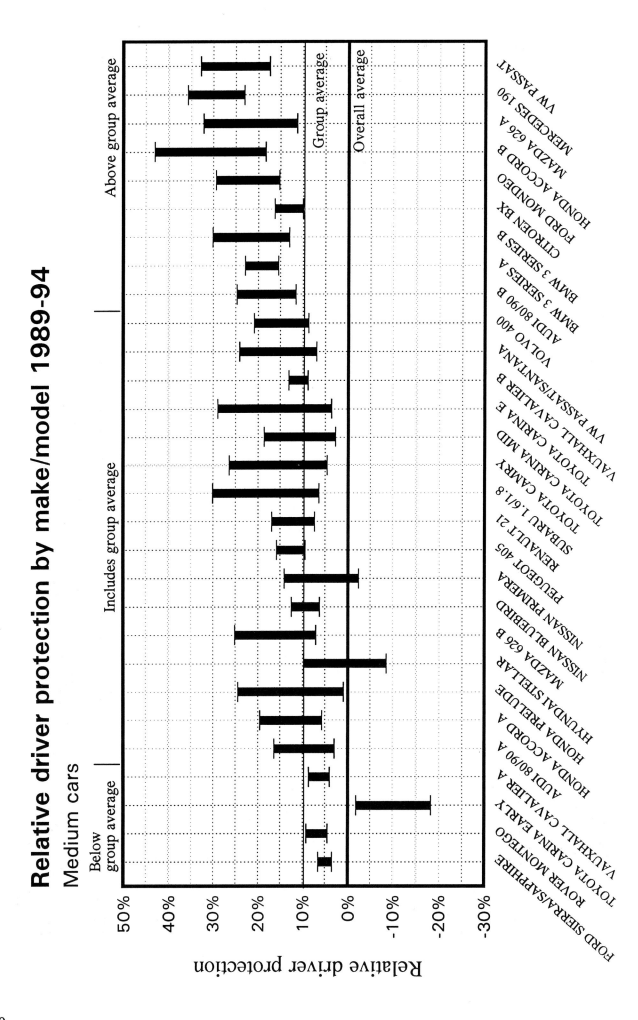

Relative driver protection by make/model 1989-94
Large cars

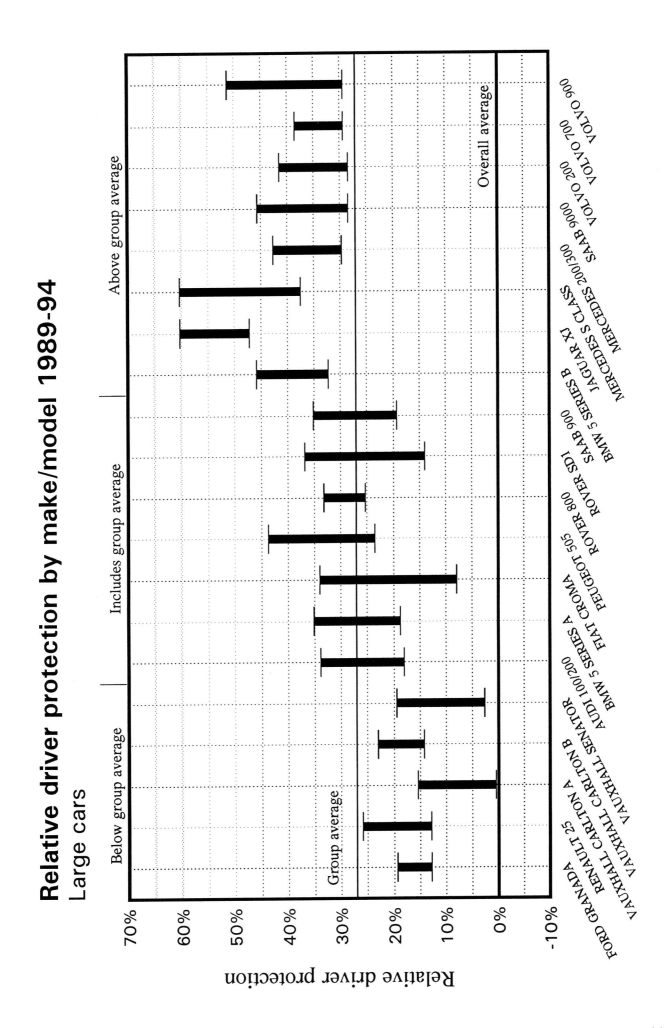

Table A Risk of injury to car drivers involved in two car injury accidents: by size and make/model of car: 1989 to 1994

		Percentage of drivers injured when involved in an injury accident [1]					
		Injury severity					
		Fatal or serious			All		
Car size/model [2]	Registration dates	Corrected [3]	95% C.I. [4]	Uncorrected	Corrected [3]	95% C.I. [4]	Uncorrected
SMALL							
CITROEN 2CV/DYANE	Jan 85 - Jul 90 [5]	11	[8 , 14]	(12)	85	[80 , 88]	(86)
CITROEN AX	Jun 87 - Dec 94	8	[7 , 9]	(8)	74	[72 , 76]	(75)
CITROEN VISA	Jan 85 - Jul 88 [5]	11	[8 , 15]	(13)	71	[65 , 77]	(74)
FIAT 126	Jan 85 - Dec 92	11	[7 , 16]	(10)	75	[67 , 81]	(81)
FIAT PANDA	Jan 85 - Dec 94	9	[8 , 11]	(9)	74	[71 , 76]	(77)
FIAT UNO	Jan 85 - Dec 94	8	[7 , 9]	(7)	69	[67 , 71]	(69)
FORD FIESTA	Jan 85 - Mar 89	8	[8 , 9]	(8)	71	[70 , 72]	(73)
FORD FIESTA	Apr 89 - Dec 94	7	[6 , 7]	(6)	70	[69 , 72]	(72)
NISSAN MICRA	Jan 85 - Dec 92	9	[8 , 10]	(8)	74	[72 , 75]	(77)
NISSAN MICRA	Jan 93 - Dec 94	10	[6 , 15]	(10)	64	[57 , 71]	(66)
PEUGEOT 106	Oct 91 - Dec 94	7	[5 , 10]	(7)	71	[66 , 75]	(73)
PEUGEOT 205	Jan 85 - Dec 94	8	[7 , 9]	(8)	67	[66 , 69]	(69)
RENAULT 5	Feb 85 - Dec 94	8	[7 , 9]	(8)	70	[68 , 72]	(71)
RENAULT CLIO	Mar 91 - Dec 94	7	[5 , 9]	(7)	65	[61 , 69]	(69)
ROVER METRO	Jan 85 - Mar 90	8	[7 , 9]	(8)	71	[70 , 72]	(74)
ROVER METRO	Apr 90 - Dec 94	8	[7 , 9]	(8)	69	[67 , 72]	(71)
ROVER MINI	Jan 85 - Dec 94	10	[9 , 12]	(10)	77	[75 , 79]	(81)
VAUXHALL CORSA	Mar 93 - Dec 94	8	[5 , 11]	(7)	66	[60 , 71]	(70)
VAUXHALL NOVA	Jan 85 - Mar 93	7	[7 , 8]	(7)	70	[69 , 72]	(73)
VOLKSWAGEN POLO	Jan 85 - Aug 94	7	[6 , 8]	(8)	70	[68 , 72]	(73)
YUGO 3/4/500	Jan 85 - Dec 91	13	[8 , 19]	(12)	64	[56 , 72]	(64)
YUGO TEMPO	Jan 85 - Dec 93	6	[4 , 9]	(5)	72	[67 , 76]	(73)
ALL SMALL		*8*		(*8*)	*71*		(*73*)
SMALL/MEDIUM							
ALFA ROMEO 33	Jan 85 - Dec 94	8	[5 , 12]	(9)	68	[60 , 74]	(63)
CITROEN ZX	Jun 91 - Dec 94	6	[4 , 8]	(6)	55	[50 , 60]	(56)
FIAT STRADA/REGATA	Jan 85 - Jun 88 [5]	8	[6 , 11]	(8)	65	[60 , 69]	(60)
FIAT TIPO/TEMPRA	Jul 88 - Dec 94	5	[4 , 7]	(5)	59	[55 , 63]	(57)
FORD ESCORT/ORION	Jan 85 - Aug 90	7	[7 , 8]	(7)	65	[64 , 65]	(62)
FORD ESCORT/ORION	Sep 90 - Dec 94	5	[5 , 6]	(5)	60	[59 , 62]	(57)
HYUNDAI PONY	Oct 85 - Aug 90	9	[7 , 13]	(10)	65	[59 , 70]	(65)
LADA RIVA [6]	Jan 85 - Dec 94	7	[6 , 9]	(8)	63	[60 , 66]	(60)
LADA SAMARA	Nov 87 - Dec 94	6	[4 , 9]	(7)	65	[61 , 69]	(63)
LANCIA DELTA/PRISMA	Jan 85 - Jul 94	10	[6 , 15]	(10)	57	[49 , 64]	(51)
MAZDA 323	Sep 85 - Sep 89	7	[5 , 9]	(7)	65	[60 , 70]	(66)
MAZDA 323	Oct 89 - Jul 94	5	[3 , 9]	(6)	61	[55 , 67]	(63)
NISSAN CHERRY	Jan 85 - Aug 86 [5]	10	[8 , 14]	(10)	72	[68 , 76]	(71)
NISSAN SUNNY	Jan 85 - Aug 86	7	[5 , 9]	(6)	67	[64 , 71]	(65)
NISSAN SUNNY	Sep 86 - Jan 91	6	[5 , 7]	(6)	63	[61 , 65]	(62)
NISSAN SUNNY	Feb 91 - Dec 94	6	[4 , 10]	(6)	63	[56 , 69]	(63)
PEUGEOT 305	Jan 85 - Jul 88 [5]	6	[4 , 9]	(8)	58	[52 , 63]	(54)
PEUGEOT 306	Apr 93 - Dec 94	4	[2 , 7]	(5)	54	[46 , 61]	(52)
PEUGEOT 309	Feb 86 - Mar 93	8	[7 , 9]	(8)	67	[65 , 68]	(65)
PROTON 1.3/1.5	Mar 89 - Dec 94	7	[5 , 10]	(8)	66	[62 , 71]	(66)
RENAULT 19	Feb 89 - Dec 94	6	[4 , 7]	(6)	60	[56 , 63]	(57)
RENAULT 9/11	Jan 85 - Jan 89 [5]	7	[6 , 9]	(7)	60	[57 , 63]	(60)
ROVER 200	Jan 85 - Sep 89	7	[7 , 8]	(8)	65	[63 , 66]	(62)
ROVER 200/400	Oct 89 - Dec 94	6	[5 , 7]	(7)	58	[56 , 60]	(55)
ROVER MAESTRO	Jan 85 - Dec 94	6	[5 , 7]	(6)	63	[61 , 64]	(60)
SEAT IBIZA/MALAGA	Oct 85 - Sep 93	6	[4 , 8]	(6)	64	[60 , 68]	(65)
SKODA ESTELLE	Jan 85 - Jul 90 [5]	8	[6 , 11]	(9)	68	[64 , 72]	(69)
SKODA FAVORIT	Jun 89 - Dec 94	7	[5 , 11]	(9)	65	[58 , 71]	(65)
TOYOTA COROLLA	Jan 85 - Aug 87	8	[6 , 10]	(7)	60	[56 , 64]	(59)
TOYOTA COROLLA	Sep 87 - Jul 92	7	[5 , 9]	(7)	62	[58 , 65]	(62)
VAUXHALL ASTRA/BELMONT	Jan 85 - Sep 91	7	[6 , 7]	(6)	63	[62 , 64]	(60)
VAUXHALL ASTRA	Oct 91 - Dec 94	4	[3 , 5]	(4)	58	[55 , 61]	(56)
VOLKSWAGEN GOLF MK1/CABRIO	Jan 85 - Dec 93	5	[4 , 7]	(5)	55	[50 , 59]	(54)
VOLKSWAGEN GOLF/JETTA	Jan 85 - Jan 92	6	[5 , 7]	(6)	59	[57 , 61]	(58)
VOLKSWAGEN GOLF/VENTO	Feb 92 - Dec 94	5	[3 , 7]	(5)	53	[48 , 58]	(53)
VOLVO 300	Jan 85 - Dec 91 [5]	5	[4 , 6]	(6)	55	[53 , 57]	(57)
ALL SMALL/MEDIUM		*7*		(*7*)	*62*		(*60*)

1 Excluding accidents in which neither driver was injured.
2 Models are listed under the current market name of the manufacturer.
3 Corrected for selected accident circumstances such as road type and driver age. Uncorrected rates are shown in brackets.
4 The probability is 95% that the true rate lies within this range.
5 Approximate withdrawal date. All cars registered up to December 1994 are included.
6 Includes earlier 1200, 1300, 1500 and 1600 models.

Table A (cont'd) Risk of injury to car drivers involved in two car injury accidents: by size and make/model of car: 1989 to 1994

Percentage of drivers injured when involved in an injury accident [1]

Car size/model [2]	Registration dates	Injury severity					
		Fatal or serious			All		
		Corrected [3]	95% C.I. [4]	Uncorrected	Corrected [3]	95% C.I. [4]	Uncorrected
MEDIUM							
AUDI 80/90	Jan 85 - Oct 86	6	[5 , 9]	(6)	57	[52 , 61]	(53)
AUDI 80/90	Nov 86 - Dec 94	4	[3 , 6]	(5)	51	[47 , 55]	(50)
BMW 3 SERIES	Jan 85 - Mar 91	6	[5 , 7]	(6)	51	[48 , 53]	(48)
BMW 3 SERIES	Apr 91 - Dec 94	4	[2 , 6]	(4)	49	[44 , 54]	(46)
CITROEN BX	Jan 85 - Dec 93 [5]	5	[4 , 6]	(6)	54	[52 , 56]	(50)
FORD MONDEO	Mar 93 - Dec 94	3	[2 , 5]	(3)	49	[44 , 53]	(44)
FORD SIERRA/SAPPHIRE	Jan 85 - Feb 93	6	[6 , 7]	(6)	59	[59 , 60]	(54)
HONDA ACCORD	Oct 85 - Sep 91	7	[5 , 10]	(7)	55	[50 , 59]	(53)
HONDA ACCORD	Oct 91 - Jul 94	2	[1 , 6]	(3)	43	[36 , 51]	(43)
HONDA PRELUDE	Jan 85 - Mar 92	5	[3 , 8]	(5)	55	[47 , 62]	(55)
HYUNDAI STELLAR	Jan 85 - Dec 91	6	[4 , 10]	(6)	62	[56 , 68]	(58)
MAZDA 626	Jan 85 - Sep 87	3	[2 , 7]	(3)	49	[42 , 56]	(46)
MAZDA 626	Oct 87 - Jan 92	7	[5 , 10]	(8)	53	[47 , 58]	(51)
MERCEDES 190	Jan 85 - Sep 93	4	[3 , 6]	(4)	44	[40 , 48]	(41)
NISSAN BLUEBIRD	Mar 86 - Aug 90 [5]	6	[5 , 7]	(5)	57	[55 , 59]	(51)
NISSAN PRIMERA	Sep 90 - Dec 94	5	[3 , 8]	(5)	59	[54 , 64]	(56)
PEUGEOT 405	Jan 88 - Dec 94	5	[5 , 6]	(6)	55	[53 , 57]	(51)
RENAULT 21	Jun 86 - Mar 94	6	[5 , 8]	(7)	55	[52 , 58]	(52)
ROVER MONTEGO	Jan 85 - Dec 94	6	[6 , 7]	(6)	58	[57 , 60]	(53)
SUBARU 1.6/1.8	Jan 85 - Dec 91	5	[3 , 8]	(7)	51	[44 , 59]	(55)
TOYOTA CAMRY	Jan 85 - Dec 86	7	[4 , 11]	(8)	53	[46 , 60]	(48)
TOYOTA CARINA	Jan 85 - Feb 88	6	[4 , 9]	(5)	69	[64 , 74]	(64)
TOYOTA CARINA	Mar 88 - Apr 92	5	[3 , 7]	(6)	56	[51 , 61]	(53)
TOYOTA CARINA E	May 92 - Dec 94	5	[2 , 9]	(4)	52	[45 , 60]	(48)
VAUXHALL CAVALIER	Jan 85 - Sep 88	6	[6 , 7]	(6)	59	[57 , 60]	(53)
VAUXHALL CAVALIER	Oct 88 - Dec 94	5	[5 , 6]	(5)	56	[54 , 57]	(51)
VOLKSWAGEN PASSAT/SANTANA	Jan 85 - May 88	6	[4 , 8]	(7)	53	[48 , 58]	(53)
VOLKSWAGEN PASSAT	Jun 88 - Dec 94	4	[3 , 6]	(5)	47	[42 , 52]	(43)
VOLVO 400	Jun 87 - Dec 94	5	[4 , 7]	(6)	53	[50 , 57]	(55)
ALL MEDIUM		*6*		(*6*)	*57*		(*52*)
LARGE							
AUDI 100/200	Jan 85 - Dec 94	3	[2 , 5]	(5)	46	[41 , 51]	(43)
BMW 5 SERIES	Jan 85 - May 88	4	[2 , 6]	(4)	46	[41 , 51]	(44)
BMW 5 SERIES	Jun 88 - Dec 94	4	[3 , 6]	(4)	38	[34 , 42]	(33)
FIAT CROMA	Jun 86 - Dec 93 [5]	8	[5 , 13]	(8)	49	[41 , 58]	(45)
FORD GRANADA	May 85 - Dec 94	6	[5 , 7]	(6)	53	[50 , 55]	(48)
JAGUAR XJ	Oct 86 - Dec 94	3	[2 , 5]	(3)	29	[25 , 33]	(27)
MERCEDES S CLASS	Jan 85 - Sep 91	4	[2 , 8]	(4)	32	[25 , 39]	(28)
MERCEDES 200/300	Oct 85 - Dec 94	4	[3 , 6]	(4)	40	[36 , 44]	(39)
PEUGEOT 505	Jan 85 - Dec 91 [5]	3	[1 , 5]	(3)	41	[35 , 48]	(42)
RENAULT 25	Jan 85 - Jan 93	5	[4 , 7]	(5)	50	[46 , 55]	(45)
ROVER 800	Jul 86 - Dec 94	4	[3 , 5]	(4)	44	[42 , 47]	(39)
ROVER SD1	Jan 85 - Jun 86 [5]	5	[3 , 9]	(5)	47	[40 , 54]	(44)
SAAB 900	Jan 85 - Sep 93	4	[3 , 6]	(5)	46	[41 , 51]	(43)
SAAB 9000	Oct 85 - Dec 94	4	[2 , 6]	(4)	39	[34 , 45]	(38)
VAUXHALL CARLTON	Jan 85 - Oct 86	6	[4 , 8]	(5)	58	[53 , 62]	(53)
VAUXHALL CARLTON	Nov 86 - Mar 94	5	[4 , 6]	(5)	51	[48 , 54]	(47)
VAUXHALL SENATOR	Sep 87 - Mar 94	5	[3 , 7]	(5)	56	[50 , 61]	(50)
VOLVO 200	Jan 85 - Dec 94	3	[2 , 5]	(4)	41	[37 , 45]	(41)
VOLVO 700	Jan 85 - Jul 91 [5]	3	[3 , 4]	(4)	41	[39 , 44]	(39)
VOLVO 900	Oct 90 - Dec 94	4	[2 , 7]	(4)	37	[31 , 44]	(37)
ALL LARGE		*4*		(*5*)	*46*		(*42*)
ALL SIZES		**7**		(**7**)	**63**		(**60**)

1 Excluding accidents in which neither driver was injured.
2 Models are listed under the current market name of the manufacturer.
3 Corrected for selected accident circumstances such as road type and driver age. Uncorrected rates are shown in brackets.
4 The probability is 95% that the true rate lies within this range.
5 Approximate withdrawal date. All cars registered up to December 1994 are included.

Table B : Description

1.26   The effects of various accident characteristics on the risk of driver injury when involved in a two car injury accident are shown in Table B. The percentages are derived using a statistical modelling technique. The most important consequence of analysing the data in this way is that the estimates of injury risk are independent of each other. For example, the estimates of injury risk on different road types are the best available estimates of the specific effect of road type, after the influences of variations in the other effects listed have been removed. The risks shown in the table relate to the average specific effects of those factors in injury accidents. Further explanation and information on the analyses are given in Appendix 3.

1.27   Table A shows the percentage of car drivers injured when involved in an injury accident for individual models of car. The percentages are derived from statistical models similar to those used for Table B but extended to allow for the effect of model of car.

Table B : Commentary

1.28   The rates shown relate to the average specific effects of those factors in injury accidents, after correcting for the influences of variations in the other factors listed. For example, the risks of injury tabulated for different sizes of car are corrected to allow for differences in the age and sex of their drivers.

1.29   Of the factors considered, those having the most influence on the risk of death or serious injury when involved in an injury accident are the speed limit of the road, the first point of impact and driver age. The most severe accidents occur on 60 mph roads, where the risk of death or serious injury to the driver is 3 times higher than on a 20 or 30 mph road. The risk of death or serious injury is about one quarter lower on a 70 mph road than on a 60 mph road, which is perhaps a reflection of the improved segregation of traffic on multi-carriageway roads. A driver is about three times more likely to be killed or seriously injured in a frontal or side impact collision than when their car is hit from behind. However a rear impact is more likely to result in slight injuries; these are likely to be whiplash neck injuries associated with either poorly adjusted or non-existent head restraints.

1.30   Age is not a large influence on the overall risk of injury when involved in an accident, although there is increased susceptibility to death or serious injury in the over 55 age group. Women are less likely to be killed when involved in an accident, which may indicate involvement at lower impact speeds. However they are about 40 per cent more likely to be injured when involved in a two car accident than men. This could be due to the different size of women, and the fact that women are more likely to sit closer to the steering wheel making them more prone to injury.

Table B   Risk of injury to drivers involved in two car injury accidents: by various factors: 1989 to 1994

| | Percentage of drivers injured when involved in a two car injury accident [1] | | |
| | Injury severity [2] | | |
Factor	Fatal	Fatal or Serious	All
Speed limit of road			
20 or 30	0.1	5	60
40 or 50	0.6	8	61
60	1.9	15	71
70	1.9	11	60
Sex of driver			
Male	0.4	7	54
Female	0.3	7	75
Age of driver			
17-24	0.3	7	63
25-34	0.3	6	62
35-54	0.4	7	62
55 or more	0.9	10	67
Size group of car			
Small	0.5	9	72
Small/medium	0.4	7	63
Medium	0.3	6	56
Large	0.2	5	46
First point of impact			
Front	0.4	8	53
Back	0.1	3	84
Offside	0.7	9	70
Nearside	0.8	8	64
All accidents	0.4	7	63

1   Excluding accidents in which neither driver was injured

2   Corrected for influences of variations in the other factors listed.

Summary

1.31   The risks of driver injury in injury accidents for particular popular models of car are presented as rates or proportions of driver injuries in Table A. The rates reflect the secondary protection offered to the driver, but also reflect the influence of mass in collisions. A problem in comparing rates, to assess the relative secondary safety of cars, is the influence of variability in accident severity. In each collision the relative severity of accident for each vehicle depends on the differences in mass between the vehicles, and also the type of accident and drivers involved. The variation in risk of driver injury due to the latter influences is accounted for by a modelling procedure which suggests that only minor adjustments should be made to the risks of driver injury in each model of car.

1.32   The assumption that each model of car has a similar distribution of collisions in terms of the size of the other car involved implies that each car is effectively being assessed against a car of average mass. Any variation in driver injury risk due to differences in the size distribution of two car collisions is therefore likely to be minimal. The ratings in Table A retain the influence of mass, and support the indication that heavier cars tend to be safer cars for their occupants. However, within size groups where car mass is less variable, there are discernible differences in risk of driver injury. It is also clear that heavier cars tend to increase the risk of injury in the cars they collide with and this is described further in Part 3.

1.33   The estimation of injury risk, and derivative car safety ratings, from road accident injury data is inevitably an evolutionary process. Methods of analysis are not static, and the amount of accident data available for a particular model of car gradually accumulates while a model is still active on the roads. Nevertheless the data records used to date do highlight some vehicles which are statistically better or worse than others, and provide some indication of relative safety. The data are recognised as a useful tool for informing car consumers about the safety features of cars, and for promoting the importance of car safety as a means of saving lives and avoiding serious injury.

PART 2

PRIMARY CAR SAFETY (Tables C and D)

Measuring Primary Car Safety

2.1   The risk of being involved in accidents is influenced mainly by driver behaviour, because the vast majority of accidents are initiated by driver error. However, vehicle characteristics such as braking, handling, lighting and drivers' fields of vision, known as primary safety factors, can influence the effects of driver error on accident risk, as can the road and traffic management infrastructure. In addition to these factors, the number of road injury accidents involving a particular type of vehicle will depend on the number of such vehicles on the road and the average mileage driven. These influences are known collectively as measures of exposure. Part 2 examines the involvement and casualty rates of different groups of car in injury accidents but the data do not fully account for exposure.

2.2   The Department obtains information on vehicle populations through analysis of Driver and Vehicle Licensing Agency (DVLA) registrations data. Quarterly vehicle stock data from DVLA are used to estimate average stock over the year for use in Tables C and D (see Appendix 5).

2.3   The accident involvement and car user casualty rates in this section are given per 10,000 licensed vehicles in each group. General information on the drivers and average mileage covered by different types of car is available from the National Travel Survey and is summarised in Appendix 6. This shows that company cars record higher mileages than privately owned cars, and that newer cars record higher mileages than older cars.

2.4   The reliability of each accident involvement and casualty rate presented in Part 2 depends on the number of licensed cars in that category. For this reason, the rates are not quoted for car types with populations of less than 20,000 licensed vehicles.

Table C : Description

2.5   Table C shows the extent to which drivers and their cars become involved in injury accidents. This is influenced mainly by driver behaviour, average mileage and pattern of use. The safety characteristics of the car will also have some influence but this is difficult to assess.

2.6   The table shows rates of involvement in injury accidents per 10,000 licensed vehicles in each of a number of groups. All injury accident involvements are included, regardless of whether the injured person was inside the car or not. Information is shown by size of car, private or company ownership, age of car, and by severity of injury.

2.7   The purpose is to illustrate differences in the rate of involvement in injury accidents for different groups of car. General information on car use, by age of car, engine capacity and ownership, extracted from the National Travel Survey, is summarised in Appendix 6.

Table C : Commentary

2.8   It is important to remember that differences in rates between groups in Table C will strongly reflect differences in the level and type of use and of driver behaviour, and should be interpreted carefully. The table shows the following:

-       Drivers of new privately owned cars are involved in less accidents than drivers of new company owned cars. This may largely be explained by the National Travel Survey data which shows that in general company owned cars record higher mileages than privately owned cars.

-       Drivers of old privately owned high performance cars have higher rates of involvement in injury accidents than drivers of their standard performance counterparts.

-       This distinction is much less clear for new cars, and for old company owned cars the standard and high performance cars have very similar involvement rates.

-       Newer private cars are seen to have lower rates of involvement in injury accidents than older cars, despite the evidence in Appendix 6 which shows that newer cars on average cover more miles each year.

Table D : Description

2.9   Table D shows car user casualty rates, which are influenced by the combined effects of accident involvement, accident type, the number of passengers and secondary safety features.

2.10   The table shows car user casualty rates per 10,000 licensed vehicles. Only persons injured while travelling inside the car are included in these rates. Information is shown by size of car, private or company ownership, and by severity of injury to occupant.

2.11   The average number of passengers carried has a much greater influence on the rates presented in Table D. However the accident reporting system does not require the police to record the number of uninjured passengers, so it is difficult to assess the size of this influence on the figures presented.

Table D : Commentary

2.12   Again, interpretation of the figures in this table depends on the relative mileages of the different types of car, their patterns of use and the behaviour of their drivers. The table shows the following:

-       In most groups about 9 to 13 car users are killed or seriously injured each year for every 10,000 licensed vehicles.

-       The car user casualty rates show a tendency to decline with increasing size of car.

-       Among older cars, company owned vehicles have generally lower casualty rates than privately owned vehicles.

-       Newer private cars usually have lower casualty rates than their older counterparts.

18

Table C   Rates of involvement in injury accidents: by size of car and ownership: 1994

Injury accident involvements per 10,000 licensed vehicles in each group

Age of car Performance Size	Privately owned		Company owned	
	Injury accident severity		Injury accident severity	
	Fatal or serious	All	Fatal or serious	All
Regd. on or since 1.1.92				
Standard				
Small	23	156	35	262
Small/medium	23	141	34	235
Medium	24	136	28	178
Large	22	117	24	148
All standard	23	144	30	198
High				
Small	23	143	..	..
Small/medium	29	146	28	198
Medium	29	140	35	235
All high	27	143	32	216
Registered before 1.1.92				
Standard				
Small	23	148	26	167
Small/medium	24	155	27	176
Medium	24	155	26	163
Large	20	124	19	121
All standard	23	150	25	156
High				
Small	35	197	..	..
Small/medium	33	183	28	165
Medium	26	149	24	147
All high	31	176	27	157

.. Denotes fewer than 20,000 licensed vehicles in the group.

Table D   Car user casualty rates: by size of car and ownership: 1994

Car user casualties per 10,000 licensed vehicles in each group

Age of car	Privately owned		Company owned	
Performance	Injury severity		Injury severity	
Size	Fatal or serious	All	Fatal or serious	All
Regd. on or since 1.1.92				
Standard				
Small	13	113	20	176
Small/medium	11	90	14	131
Medium	10	79	8	81
Large	9	62	6	61
All standard	12	95	11	102
High				
Small	11	88	..	..
Small/medium	11	69	11	101
Medium	7	60	10	109
All high	10	72	11	107
Registered before 1.1.92				
Standard				
Small	13	112	15	116
Small/medium	13	103	11	100
Medium	11	92	10	82
Large	7	61	7	51
All standard	12	99	10	83
High				
Small	21	142	..	..
Small/medium	20	119	14	95
Medium	13	84	9	68
All high	18	114	12	82

.. Denotes fewer than 20,000 licensed vehicles in the group.

PART 3

CAR SAFETY RATINGS: RELATED ANALYSES

The aggressivity of cars in two-car collisions

3.1   In Part 1 it was noted that although mass was beneficial to a driver in a relatively heavy car, it could be detrimental to the drivers of other cars with which it collided. It is possible to calculate ratings based on the injuries sustained by the driver of the "other car" when colliding with certain make/models. In other words to calculate the proportion of drivers in Car 2 injured in collisions with a given model of car (Car 1).

3.2   Following the nomenclature in the description of Table A on page 4, the calculation of the risk of injury as the percentage of drivers injured in a car (say car 2) when colliding with a specific model of car (car 1) can be represented as follows:

$$\frac{X_2 + X_3}{X_1 + X_2 + X_3} \times 100$$

where

X_1 = Number of accidents in which driver injured in car 1 but not in car 2
X_2 = Number of accidents in which driver injured in car 1 and in car 2
X_3 = Number of accidents in which driver injured in car 2 but not in car 1

3.3   While, in general, models which were rated as safer than their group average were found to be more aggressive, this was not exclusively the case. There were examples of models offering, say, average protection but being significantly either more or less aggressive than average. In other words, although generally, as one would expect, the ratings for aggressivity were the inverse of those for safety, there were some significant differences both across the range of models and within size groups.

3.4   Chart E plots the best estimates of the aggressivity ratings against those for the risk of injury and illustrates that the former generally correlate highly with the inverse of the latter. The chart also contains one or two outliers suggesting that some models may not adhere to this pattern; for example, there were some models which perform relatively well on at least one of the measures without necessarily having an inverse (ie. poor) rating on the other. In other words the aggregate number of injuries in collisions involving these models was less than average, suggesting that some models may strike a better balance than others between protecting their own drivers and minimising their aggressivity towards others.

Chart E The relationship between the Aggressivity and Risk of injury ratings

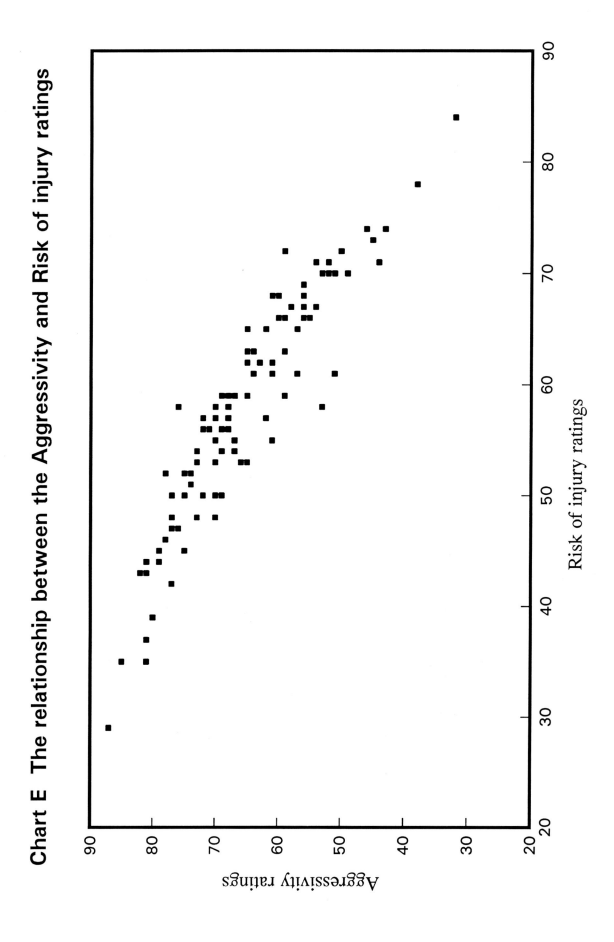

Risk of injury ratings

Aggressivity ratings

Mass-adjusted car safety ratings

3.5   From an individual driver's point of view the mass of car is certainly to be regarded as a safety factor, because the laws of physics determine that they will be safer in most accidents when they are driving a heavier or larger car. However it would be interesting to compare cars only on the basis of the secondary protection that is offered by their structure, design and secondary safety fittings. This requires a procedure to remove the influence of mass from the calculation of risk of driver injury. Initial work has been carried out to remove the specific effects of mass from the relative risks of driver injury so that relative safety ratings of car models can be made in terms of their inherent design features and secondary safety fittings. The methodology used is that described in the research work carried out by the Transport Research Laboratory and set out in their recent report (see Appendix 1).

3.6   In short, the mass adjusted ratings derived from the risk of injury are based on the difference between the unadjusted rating and the "expected" rating for a car of that mass. In theory this difference is attributable to model specific design effects. The expected rating is obtained by fitting a linear model between the risk of injury and mass for each of the car models covered in the analysis. This produced the following relationship:

"Expected" risk (per 100 accs) = 103.3 - 0.044 Mass   ($R^2 = 0.77$),
implying that for every extra 100 KG, the risk of injury (per 100 accidents) falls by 4.4.

3.7   The expected risks are then subtracted from the unadjusted risks of injury as published in Table A (ie. unadjusted for mass) to produce the Mass-adjusted Safety Index (MSI).

3.8   After mass adjustment, the pattern of larger models generally being safest no longer applies, although early indications suggest there are very few small cars among the models with the safest ratings. This may be due to the fact that a more extensive range of safety fittings are more likely to be found in larger cars than smaller cars.

3.9   An assumption lying behind all the recent car safety work, and one which is particularly important to this analysis, is that each make/model collides with a similar distribution of cars in terms of the size and, more importantly, mass of the second car involved. This was found to be true in terms of the four size groups based on length of car and we are now able to investigate whether the assumption is correct with regard to mass. Appendix 4 shows the distribution of collisions for each model and size group of car split by the mass of the collision partner and confirms that the assumption holds.

3.10   The calculation of mass adjusted safety ratings depends critically upon the quality and availability of detailed mass data for specific car models. The ratings may also be influenced by differences in passenger and luggage loading in cars. This analysis is still at a experimental stage and further progress is dependent on the extent to which the necessary mass data can be accumulated. Therefore it would not be appropriate to publish model specific ratings at this stage.

Collisions between cars and pedestrians

3.11   The following analysis is based on data from accidents involving injured pedestrians and one car in the years 1986-94. To set the analysis in context, this subset of accidents is responsible for a substantial number of casualties; in 1994 over 700 pedestrians were killed and 9000 seriously injured by cars. Casualties of all severities in 1994 in these types of accident were nearly 40,000.

3.12   Car safety analysis is based upon the proportion of drivers injured in two-car collisions. In this assessment of the aggressivity of cars and drivers towards pedestrians, all pedestrians are, by definition, injured. The approach therefore focuses on the proportions of the pedestrians that were seriously or fatally injured, and possible contributory factors.

3.13   However, a preliminary investigation of the aggressivity of younger and older car drivers can be deduced from a comparison of their pedestrian collisions in relation to their mileage driven. Table F shows the numbers and proportions of car drivers involved in collisions with pedestrians by age and sex of car driver.

3.14   The table shows that 73% of collisions between cars and pedestrians involve male drivers which broadly reflects the proportion of total car mileage driven by men. However, the data show that young drivers are involved in a disproportionately large number of collisions with pedestrians when the estimates of their mileage is taken into account. This effect is particularly strong for male drivers, where those aged between 16 and 24 account for 7 percent of mileage driven but 19 percent of collisions with pedestrians. This could be due to inexperience and lack of roadcraft. For example younger drivers, and male drivers, may drive too fast for the road conditions reducing their reaction time to dangerous traffic situations.

3.15   Table G shows the effect of various factors on the severity of injury to pedestrians hit by cars. The table shows the following:

Pedestrian age

3.16   Older pedestrians are more likely to be killed or seriously injured. This effect is most marked in the over 55 age group, where pedestrians are about one and a half times more likely than average to be seriously injured, and three times more likely to be killed.

Point of impact on car

3.17   Not surprisingly, impacts with the rear of a car are least severe, probably because in these collisions vehicles are moving slower than average. Frontal impacts on pedestrians are three times as likely to be fatal as side impacts.

Speed limit of road

3.18   Although only a proxy for speed of impact, the table predictably shows that collisions on faster roads are more severe. At the extreme, a person hit on a 70mph road is shown to have a one in five chance of being killed, over ten times the likelihood of being killed on a 30mph road.

Driver age

3.19   Driver age has no significant effect on the likelihood of a pedestrian being killed or seriously injured. The table does, however, show that pedestrians hit by cars driven by drivers in the younger age bands are most likely to be killed. This could be because younger drivers drive at inappropriate speeds in urban areas, the net effect of which is to relatively increase both the number of collisions with pedestrians (see Table F) and the relative severity of the collisions.

Driver sex

3.20   Pedestrians hit by a car with a male driver are slightly more likely to be killed or seriously injured and are about one and a half times more likely to be killed than by a car with a female driver, which may again reflect on the driving behaviour of males compared to females.

Table F Car - Pedestrian collisions and mileage driven: by age and sex of driver: 1986 to 1994

		Number of collisions	Percent	Mileage driven (%)
Male	16-24	57,951	19	7
	25-34	63,407	21	16
	35-54	72,912	24	36
	55 or more	30,922	10	14
	All ages	225,192	73	72
Female	16-24	20,436	7	3
	25-34	26,245	9	8
	35-54	29,481	10	13
	55 or more	7,222	2	3
	All ages	83,384	27	28
All drivers		308,576	100	100

1 Relates to accidents in the period 1986-94. Mileage data from National Travel Survey.

Table G Severity of injury to pedestrians hit by cars:
by selected factors: 1986 to 1994

		Percentage of injured pedestrians that are seriously or fatally injured [1]	
		Injury severity	
Factor		Fatal	Fatal or serious
Age of pedestrian	0-15	0.8	25.6
	16-24	1.1	25.7
	25-34	1.3	26.6
	35-54	2.2	30.1
	55 or more	6.0	44.5
Age of driver	16-24	2.8	34.9
	25-34	2.1	30.5
	35-54	1.8	28.2
	55 or more	1.9	28.9
Sex of driver	Male	2.4	31.3
	Female	1.5	27.4
Point of impact with car	Front	2.6	32.8
	Back	0.5	17.5
	Offside	0.9	25.7
	Nearside	0.9	24.3
Speed limit of road (mph)	20 or 30	1.6	27.8
	40 or 50	6.0	47.5
	60	7.6	51.4
	70	19.0	78.4
All car-pedestrian collisions		2.0	29.6

1 Starting point is injured pedestrians.

APPENDIX 1 BACKGROUND AND DETAILED NOTES

Introduction

By agreement between the Department of Transport and police forces throughout Great Britain, details of all road accidents reported to the police in which a person is injured are transmitted to the Department of Transport in the form of a standard report (STATS19), usually through the appropriate local authority. These accident reports provide the basis for the Department's work on monitoring and analysis of road accident statistics.

From January 1989 the standard report prepared by the police was modified to include the registration marks of all motor vehicles involved in accidents. By linking the registration marks with the vehicle data held by DVLA at Swansea, a range of extra information about the vehicles involved in injury accidents can now be obtained. No personal details, such as names or addresses, are collected in this process.

This is the sixth report of results based on these additional vehicle data. It presents estimates of injury risk to drivers involved in injury accidents for popular car models, and also injury accident rates for different types of car and the types and numbers of casualties resulting from these accidents. The first report of this type, covering accidents in 1989, was published by HMSO in May 1991.

Coverage

It is not possible to link all vehicles involved in road injury accidents with vehicle registration data at DVLA. Details of foreign, diplomatic and military vehicles and those with trade plates are not held at DVLA. In addition, registration marks are generally unavailable for vehicles which leave the scene of an accident and some registration marks which appear to have a valid format prove untraceable.

Since 1991 these factors collectively resulted in roughly 15 per cent of vehicles having no additional vehicle details. Due to the varying rates at which registration marks began to be recorded by police forces the corresponding figures for preceding years were higher than this.

The number of two car collisions analysed to produce the tables in Part 1 of this report is considerably lower than the number of two car collisions recorded in, say, the Department's annual publication Road Accidents Great Britain. This difference is due to several factors. In order to be included in the analysis it is necessary to have the vehicle registration data of **both** cars involved. Although, for the reasons outlined in the preceding paragraphs, the detailed vehicle data is available for over 80 per cent of the cars, the requirement to have data for both cars results in approximately 70 per cent of the two car accidents (as published in Road Accidents Great Britain) being included in the analysis.

The number of accidents is further reduced due to several refinements to the dataset which aim to ensure that cars are being compared on as even a basis as possible. This involves narrowing the broader definition of car that is used for other publications and excluding accidents involving parked cars. In addition the analysis is restricted to accidents in which one or both of the drivers was injured. The resultant dataset, designed to minimise variation in accident types between different car models which could unduly bias comparisons of driver injury risk in particular car models, contains approximately 45 per cent of the two car accidents published in Road Accidents Great Britain. Accident types that could otherwise bias ratings are therefore directly eliminated from the analysis. If they had been retained the relatively less powerful procedure of having to allow for their influence in a more complex modelling process would have had to be adopted.

Any bias due to missing data would be unlikely to significantly influence the ratings. It is reasonable to expect that missing data are unlikely to be concentrated in particular types of accidents for particular models of car, but are more likely to be randomly spread over all accident types and all models of car. Tests were conducted to check that the final dataset is typical of all two car collisions in terms of driver and accident characteristics. The results, shown below, demonstrate that in terms of driver sex, driver age and speed limit of road the dataset used in the secondary safety analysis is broadly representative.

Two car collisions by accident/driver type (%), 1989-94

	Road Accidents GB Table 23	Cars: Make and Model Table A
Speed limit of road		
20-39	61	58
40-59	11	12
60-69	23	24
70	5	5
Total	100	100
Driver sex		
Male	69	63
Female	31	37
Total	100	100
Driver age		
17-24	29	28
25-34	28	28
35-54	31	31
55+	13	13
Total	100	100

Other publications

Similar reports on car safety have been published in the United States of America by the Insurance Institute for Highway Safety, in Sweden by the Folksam Insurance Company, in Australia by the Monash University Accident Research Centre, in Finland by the University of Oulu and in the UK by the Transport Research Laboratory. Each produces a summary report for widespread distribution.

References:-

Insurance Institute for Highway Safety: Status Report. Vol 24, No 11.
1005 North Glebe Road, Arlington, VA 22201. ISSN 0018-988X.

Safe and Dangerous Cars 1989-90: A report from Folksam.
Folksam, Division for Research and Development, S-106 60 Stockholm.

The Effect of Driver's Age and Experience and Car Model on Accident Risk.
University of Oulu, Finland, Publications of Road and Transport Laboratory 1992.

Vehicle Crashworthiness Ratings: Victoria and NSW crashes during 1987-92. Technical Report.
Monash University Accident Research Centre, Australia, 1994.

The Theoretical Basis for Comparing the Accident Record of Car Models (Project Report 70).
Dr J Broughton, Safety Research Centre, Transport Research Laboratory 1994.

APPENDIX 2 DEFINITIONS

The statistics refer to accidents involving cars resulting in personal injury on public roads, including footways, which became known to the police. Results for 1994 include all accidents in that year determined by the date of accident. Tables in Part 1 include accidents in all years from 1989 to 1994 inclusive. Figures for deaths refer to persons who sustained injuries causing death at the time of the accident or within 30 days of the accident, which is the internationally recognised definition.

Injury severity   *Severity* of an *injury* to a casualty is determined by the degree of injury and is either *fatal*, *seriously injured* or *slightly injured*.

Accident Severity   *Severity* of an *accident*, is determined by the severity of injury of the most severely injured casualty in that accident. That is *fatal*, where one or more persons involved in the accident were killed, *serious*, where one or more persons involved were seriously injured but no-one killed, or *slight*, where one or more persons involved were slightly injured but no-one killed or seriously injured.

Car   Any four-wheeled car. This includes saloons, hatch-backs, estates, "people carriers", coupes and convertibles. Purpose-built taxis, car derived vans, goods vehicles and minibuses are not included.

Size   Not formally defined but arranged so that the consumer can recognise standard groups. As an approximate guide, cars in the *small* group are generally between 140 and 150 inches in length and broadly equate to the motor industry's "minis" and "super-minis". Those in the *small/medium* group (equal to the industry's "lower medium") are between 155 and 165 inches, those in the *medium* group (= "upper medium") between 170 and 180 inches, and those in the *large* group (= "executive" and "luxury") over 180 inches. The allocation of a particular model to a size group does not imply that the model meets any formal classification or standard.

High performance   No single criterion has been adopted for the purpose of identifying cars in this category. Models whose performance is considerably higher than the standard production range are included. Most will be fitted with engines of higher capacity than their standard performance counterparts, and may also have features such as fuel injection or be fitted with turbo chargers. Typically, though not invariably, they have the capability of accelerating from 0 to 60 mph in 10 seconds or less.

In the large group most cars are fitted with engines of greater power and higher cubic capacity. There is less distinction between standard and higher performance cars, so all cars in this size group have been classed as standard.

New and *Old* cars   Used in this report to describe cars registered on or after 1st January 1992 and before 1st January 1992 respectively. That is *new* describes cars up to three years old at the end of 1994, and *old* describes cars three years old or more at the same date.

Ownership type   Identified from the registered keeper record at DVLA. *Company* cars are registered in the name of a company or partnership. *Private* cars are registered in the name of an individual.

APPENDIX 3   EXPLANATORY NOTES TO STATISTICAL MODELLING IN TABLES A AND B

The risk of injury to a driver involved in an accident clearly depends on a range of factors. Table B shows that the age and sex of driver, the speed of road and point of impact can all effect the risk of injury.

Valid comparisons of the inherent secondary safety records of different models of car are therefore complicated. Involvement in a high proportion of accidents with a low risk of driver injury will tend to produce a better apparent safety record whereas involvement in a high proportion of accidents with a high risk of driver injury will tend to produce a worse apparent safety record.

In order to isolate individual influences, statistical modelling has been used, which works by imagining that the risk of injury depends on a range of factors. The models look at the influences on the logarithm of the odds of injury, sometimes called the logit function, rather than directly at the influences on the proportion of accidents resulting in injury. This technique, known as logistic regression or logistic analysis, allows the influences on the risk of injury to be isolated and treated in an additive way. Unfortunately, the resulting factors are difficult to interpret by a non-specialist readership, so they have therefore been used to calculate corrected estimates of the percentage of drivers injured.

The statistical analyses used for Table B form the basis for the make/model comparisons in Table A. The largest influences on risk of injury to the driver in an accident identified from the statistical models used for Table B are also included in the statistical analyses comparing models of car used for Table A. The results are the best available estimates of the underlying secondary safety record, corrected for differences in key accident circumstances that influence the risk of injury to the driver.

The reliability of the result for a model of car in Table A depends on the number of recorded accident involvements of that model. Only those models exceeding the threshold of 150 involvements are included. In order to indicate the reliability of figures relating to individual models all estimates are accompanied by their associated 95 per cent confidence interval.

APPENDIX 3   EXPLANATORY NOTES TO STATISTICAL MODELLING (CONT.)

Statistical model used for each injury severity risk in Table A:

$$Y_{jklmn} = \mu + B_j + C_k + D_l + E_m + M_n + \varepsilon_{jklmn},$$

where $Y_{jklmn} = \text{Log}_e \left[P_{jklmn}/(1-P_{jklmn}) \right]$

and $P_{jklmn} = n_{jklmn}/N_{jklmn},$

where $N_{jklmn} = $ Number of drivers in group $_{jklmn}$

and $n_{jklmn} = $ Number of injured drivers in group $_{jklmn},$

and where the effects are represented by: -

μ Overall mean,

B_j Speed limit of road,

C_k First point of impact,

D_l Sex of driver,

E_m Age group of driver,

M_n Effect for model of car, and

ε Error term.

Statistical model used for each injury severity risk in Table B:

$$Y_{ijklm} = \mu + A_i + B_j + C_k + D_l + E_m + \varepsilon_{ijklm},$$

where the effects are represented as above and by: -

A_i Size of car.

APPENDIX 4 DISTRIBUTION OF INVOLVEMENTS BY MASS OF COLLISION PARTNER

Car size/model	Registration dates	Collision partner mass group (%)										
		<600 kg	601 - 700 kg	701 - 800 kg	801 - 900 kg	901 - 1000 kg	1001 - 1100 kg	1101 - 1200 kg	1201 - 1300 kg	1301 - 1400 kg	>1400 kg	Total
SMALL												
CITROEN 2CV/DYANE	Jan 85 - Jul 90	0	0	10	27	26	21	7	1	5	2	100
CITROEN AX	Jun 87 - Dec 94	0	0	8	28	26	21	9	2	5	2	100
CITROEN VISA	Jan 85 - Jul 88	0	0	9	31	24	18	9	2	3	3	100
FIAT 126	Jan 85 - Dec 92	0	1	8	23	24	22	10	2	7	2	100
FIAT PANDA	Jan 85 - Dec 94	0	0	10	26	24	22	9	2	5	2	100
FIAT UNO	Jan 85 - Dec 94	0	0	9	27	27	21	8	1	5	2	100
FORD FIESTA	Jan 85 - Mar 89	0	0	9	27	27	19	10	2	5	2	100
FORD FIESTA	Apr 89 - Dec 94	0	0	8	27	27	18	10	2	5	2	100
NISSAN MICRA	Jan 85 - Dec 92	0	0	9	27	28	16	11	2	5	1	100
NISSAN MICRA	Jan 93 - Dec 94	1	0	9	21	31	17	14	3	4	1	100
PEUGEOT 106	Oct 91 - Dec 94	0	0	8	25	31	16	12	2	5	2	100
PEUGEOT 205	Jan 85 - Dec 94	0	0	9	26	29	16	11	2	5	2	100
RENAULT 5	Feb 85 - Dec 94	0	0	9	25	28	17	11	3	5	2	100
RENAULT CLIO	Mar 91 - Dec 94	0	0	8	26	31	16	12	3	3	2	100
ROVER METRO	Jan 85 - Mar 90	0	0	9	25	31	14	12	2	4	1	100
ROVER METRO	Apr 90 - Dec 94	0	0	9	25	31	14	11	3	5	1	100
ROVER MINI	Jan 85 - Dec 94	0	0	9	25	30	15	11	2	4	2	100
VAUXHALL CORSA	Mar 93 - Dec 94	0	0	9	28	30	10	14	4	4	1	100
VAUXHALL NOVA	Jan 85 - Mar 93	0	0	8	25	34	12	12	2	4	1	100
VW POLO	Jan 85 - Aug 94	0	0	8	25	36	13	12	3	3	1	100
YUGO 3/4/500	Jan 85 - Dec 91	1	0	10	19	38	13	10	2	5	1	100
YUGO TEMPO	Jan 85 - Dec 93	1	0	9	21	37	12	13	2	4	1	100
ALL SMALL		0	0	9	26	29	17	11	2	5	2	100
SMALL/MEDIUM												
ALFA ROMEO 33	Jan 85 - Dec 94	0	0	7	25	28	23	6	0	8	2	100
CITROEN ZX	Jun 91 - Dec 94	0	0	11	28	21	22	11	1	4	2	100
FIAT STRADA/REGATA	Jan 85 - Jun 88	0	0	10	27	25	19	8	3	5	3	100
FIAT TIPO/TEMPRA	Jul 88 - Dec 94	0	0	8	27	26	21	10	1	5	1	100
FORD ESCORT/ORION	Jan 85 - Aug 90	0	0	9	27	26	20	9	2	5	2	100
FORD ESCORT/ORION	Sep 90 - Dec 94	0	0	9	27	26	18	10	3	5	2	100
HYUNDAI PONY	Oct 85 - Aug 90	0	0	9	28	27	16	11	4	3	1	100
LADA RIVA	Jan 85 - Dec 94	0	0	11	26	27	16	12	2	5	2	100
LADA SAMARA	Nov 87 - Dec 94	0	0	9	26	27	18	12	2	5	2	100
LANCIA DELTA/PRISMA	Jan 85 - Jul 94	0	0	9	25	31	18	9	3	3	2	100
MAZDA 323	Sep 85 - Sep 89	0	0	8	28	27	17	11	3	4	1	100
MAZDA 323	Oct 89 - Jul 94	0	0	14	27	23	18	9	2	6	1	100
NISSAN CHERRY	Jan 85 - Aug 86	0	0	10	26	29	16	10	3	4	2	100
NISSAN SUNNY	Jan 85 - Aug 86	0	0	9	25	29	17	11	2	4	2	100
NISSAN SUNNY	Sep 86 - Jan 91	0	0	8	27	27	16	12	2	5	1	100
NISSAN SUNNY	Feb 91 - Dec 94	1	0	12	27	27	16	9	3	5	0	100
PEUGEOT 305	Jan 85 - Jul 88	0	0	10	29	26	13	13	2	5	2	100
PEUGEOT 306	Apr 93 - Dec 94	1	0	10	30	22	20	12	1	3	2	100
PEUGEOT 309	Feb 86 - Mar 93	0	0	8	27	30	15	10	3	5	2	100
PROTON 1.3/1.5	Mar 89 - Dec 94	0	0	7	21	32	18	13	2	6	1	100
RENAULT 19	Feb 89 - Dec 94	0	0	8	25	33	14	11	2	6	1	100
RENAULT 9/11	Jan 85 - Jan 89	0	0	8	25	29	16	12	2	5	2	100
ROVER 200	Jan 85 - Sep 89	0	0	9	26	30	15	12	2	4	2	100
ROVER 200/400	Oct 89 - Dec 94	0	0	9	26	30	16	11	2	4	1	100
ROVER MAESTRO	Jan 85 - Dec 94	0	0	9	26	30	14	11	3	5	2	100
SEAT IBIZA/MALAGA	Oct 85 - Sep 93	0	0	10	27	31	14	9	2	5	1	100
SKODA ESTELLE	Jan 85 - Jul 90	0	0	9	25	32	15	12	2	4	1	100
SKODA FAVORIT	Jun 89 - Dec 94	0	0	8	28	31	17	9	2	2	2	100
TOYOTA COROLLA	Jan 85 - Aug 87	0	0	9	26	33	15	10	2	3	1	100
TOYOTA COROLLA	Sep 87 - Jul 92	0	0	9	26	30	14	11	2	5	1	100
VAUXHALL ASTRA/BELMONT	Jan 85 - Sep 91	0	0	9	25	32	13	12	3	4	2	100
VAUXHALL ASTRA	Oct 91 - Dec 94	0	0	7	26	32	14	12	2	5	1	100
VW GOLF MK1/CABRIOLET	Jan 85 - Dec 93	0	0	8	24	34	12	13	3	4	2	100
VW GOLF/JETTA	Jan 85 - Jan 92	0	0	10	24	33	12	13	3	4	1	100
VW GOLF/VENTO	Feb 92 - Dec 94	0	0	7	29	30	12	13	2	5	1	100
VOLVO 300	Jan 85 - Dec 91	0	0	10	24	35	11	13	2	4	1	100
ALL SMALL/MEDIUM		0	0	9	26	29	16	11	2	5	2	100

APPENDIX 4 DISTRIBUTION OF INVOLVEMENTS BY MASS OF COLLISION PARTNER (CONT.)

| Car size/model | Registration dates | Collision partner mass group (%) | | | | | | | | | | |
		<600 kg	601 - 700 kg	701 - 800 kg	801 - 900 kg	901 - 1000 kg	1001 - 1100 kg	1101 - 1200 kg	1201 - 1300 kg	1301 - 1400 kg	>1400 kg	Total
MEDIUM												
AUDI 80/90	Jan 85 - Oct 86	0	0	10	27	24	21	6	2	7	2	100
AUDI 80/90	Nov 86 - Dec 94	0	0	10	28	23	20	9	2	6	2	100
BMW 3 SERIES	Jan 85 - Mar 91	0	0	10	26	25	21	8	2	6	2	100
BMW 3 SERIES	Apr 91 - Dec 94	0	0	7	29	29	17	11	2	3	2	100
CITROEN BX	Jan 85 - Dec 93	0	0	9	27	23	22	10	2	6	2	100
FORD MONDEO	Mar 93 - Dec 94	0	0	10	25	30	16	10	3	5	1	100
FORD SIERRA/SAPPHIRE	Jan 85 - Feb 93	0	0	9	26	28	17	11	2	5	2	100
HONDA ACCORD	Oct 85 - Sep 91	0	0	7	27	26	16	12	3	7	2	100
HONDA ACCORD	Oct 91 - Jul 94	0	0	6	24	33	18	11	3	4	2	100
HONDA PRELUDE	Jan 85 - Mar 92	0	0	6	22	26	21	13	5	6	1	100
MAZDA 626	Jan 85 - Sep 87	0	0	10	26	29	16	9	2	6	2	100
MAZDA 626	Oct 87 - Jan 92	0	0	10	24	30	18	10	3	4	2	100
MERCEDES 190	Jan 85 - Sep 93	0	0	10	24	29	18	9	3	5	3	100
NISSAN BLUEBIRD	Mar 86 - Aug 90	0	0	9	27	29	15	11	2	4	2	100
NISSAN PRIMERA	Sep 90 - Dec 94	0	0	12	23	29	16	13	1	5	0	100
PEUGEOT 405	Jan 88 - Dec 94	0	0	8	26	30	15	11	3	5	2	100
RENAULT 21	Jun 86 - Mar 94	0	0	9	23	31	17	11	2	5	1	100
ROVER MONTEGO	Jan 85 - Dec 94	0	0	9	25	31	14	11	2	5	1	100
SUBARU 1.6/1.8	Jan 85 - Dec 91	1	0	11	24	31	13	10	3	5	2	100
TOYOTA CAMRY	Jan 85 - Dec 86	0	0	11	27	30	13	12	4	3	1	100
TOYOTA CARINA	Jan 85 - Feb 88	0	0	9	21	37	13	14	3	2	1	100
TOYOTA CARINA	Mar 88 - Apr 92	0	0	7	25	33	15	13	2	4	1	100
TOYOTA CARINA E	May 92 - Dec 94	0	0	3	26	33	17	15	4	2	2	100
VAUXHALL CAVALIER	Jan 85 - Sep 88	0	0	9	25	32	12	12	3	4	1	100
VAUXHALL CAVALIER	Oct 88 - Dec 94	0	0	9	25	32	12	13	3	4	1	100
VW PASSAT/SANTANA	Jan 85 - May 88	1	0	9	24	33	12	13	2	4	2	100
VW PASSAT	Jun 88 - Dec 94	0	0	9	26	30	12	11	3	4	2	100
VOLVO 400	Jun 87 - Dec 94	1	0	9	25	33	11	14	3	3	1	100
ALL MEDIUM		0	0	9	25	30	16	11	2	5	2	100
LARGE												
AUDI 100/200	Jan 85 - Dec 94	0	0	9	28	22	25	7	2	4	2	100
BMW 5 SERIES	Jan 85 - May 88	0	0	10	25	24	23	8	2	6	2	100
BMW 5 SERIES	Jun 88 - Dec 94	0	0	11	25	25	22	9	1	5	2	100
FIAT CROMA	Jun 86 - Dec 93	0	0	8	24	22	22	14	1	7	2	100
FORD GRANADA	May 85 - Dec 94	0	0	8	26	27	20	11	2	5	2	100
JAGUAR XJ	Oct 86 - Dec 94	0	0	9	29	27	17	9	2	5	2	100
MERCEDES S CLASS	Jan 85 - Sep 91	0	0	9	29	30	13	10	3	3	2	100
MERCEDES 200/300	Oct 85 - Dec 94	0	0	11	26	25	17	12	3	3	3	100
PEUGEOT 505	Jan 85 - Dec 91	0	0	8	26	25	22	10	1	5	3	100
RENAULT 25	Jan 85 - Jan 93	0	0	9	27	26	16	14	2	4	2	100
ROVER 800	Jul 86 - Dec 94	0	0	8	27	30	15	11	2	4	2	100
ROVER SD1	Jan 85 - Jun 86	0	0	9	25	33	13	10	3	5	1	100
SAAB 900	Jan 85 - Sep 93	1	0	10	24	32	15	11	3	4	1	100
SAAB 9000	Oct 85 - Dec 94	0	0	10	21	37	14	11	1	4	2	100
VAUXHALL CARLTON	Jan 85 - Oct 86	0	0	8	25	31	13	11	4	5	2	100
VAUXHALL CARLTON	Nov 86 - Mar 94	0	0	8	23	35	14	13	2	4	1	100
VAUXHALL SENATOR	Sep 87 - Mar 94	0	0	7	24	35	11	14	3	4	2	100
VOLVO 200	Jan 85 - Dec 94	0	0	9	23	35	13	14	2	4	1	100
VOLVO 700	Jan 85 - Jul 91	0	0	8	21	37	10	15	3	4	1	100
VOLVO 900	Oct 90 - Dec 94	1	1	6	19	38	11	15	3	6	1	100
ALL LARGE		0	0	9	25	30	16	12	2	5	2	100
ALL SIZES		0	0	9	26	29	16	11	2	5	2	100

35

APPENDIX 5   ADJUSTMENTS TO 1994 STOCK FIGURES USED IN PART 2

In this publication, the annual average stock data used in tables C and D have been calculated using quarterly stock figures, as follows:

$$\text{annual average stock} = \frac{\text{1 Jan 94 stock}}{10} + \frac{2(\text{31 Mar 94 stock} + \text{30 Jun 94 stock} + \text{30 Sep 94 stock})}{10} + \frac{\text{31 Dec 94 stock}}{10}$$

In previous publications quarterly data were unavailable, so the annual average stock had to be estimated from end year stock using a separate factor for each of new privately owned cars, new company cars, old privately owned cars and old company cars. When these factors were applied to end 1994 stock figures the results were found to be very similar to those produced using the quarterly data, but it must be borne in mind that the stock figures used in this publication are not exactly comparable with those used in earlier years.

APPENDIX 6   INFORMATION ON AVERAGE MILEAGE DRAWN FROM THE NATIONAL TRAVEL SURVEY 1992-94

1.   Estimated annual average mileage of four wheeled cars, by age and ownership of car, 1992-94

	Company	Private
Up to 1 year old	22,000	10,200
Over 1 and up to 2 years old	23,000	10,000
Over 2 and up to 3 years old	21,200	9,900
Over 3 years old	17,700	8,100
All ages	20,800	8,600

2.   Estimated annual average mileage of four wheeled cars, by engine capacity of car, 1992-94

Up to 1000 cc	5,600
1001 to 1300 cc	7,600
1301 to 1400 cc	9,500
1401 to 1800 cc	11,000
1801 to 2000 cc	12,800
2001 cc or more	12,100
All capacities	9,500

Printed in the United Kingdom for HMSO
Dd 0301513   C5   10/95   3396   17434   336130